1 MONTH OF FREE READING

at

www.ForgottenBooks.com

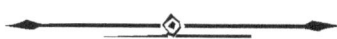

By purchasing this book you are eligible for one month membership to ForgottenBooks.com, giving you unlimited access to our entire collection of over 700,000 titles via our web site and mobile apps.

To claim your free month visit:

www.forgottenbooks.com/free820739

* Offer is valid for 45 days from date of purchase. Terms and conditions apply.

ISBN 978-0-332-09646-9
PIBN 10820739

This book is a reproduction of an important historical work. Forgotten Books uses state-of-the-art technology to digitally reconstruct the work, preserving the original format whilst repairing imperfections present in the aged copy. In rare cases, an imperfection in the original, such as a blemish or missing page, may be replicated in our edition. We do, however, repair the vast majority of imperfections successfully; any imperfections that remain are intentionally left to preserve the state of such historical works.

Forgotten Books is a registered trademark of FB &c Ltd.
Copyright © 2017 FB &c Ltd.
FB &c Ltd, Dalton House, 60 Windsor Avenue, London, SW19 2RR.
Company number 08720141. Registered in England and Wales.

For support please visit www.forgottenbooks.com

A PRE-CANE ORIENTATION & MOBILITY OUTLINE
FOR THE PARENTS AND TEACHERS OF
THE VISUALLY IMPAIRED

Prepared by
John Zimbelman
Orientation and Mobility Specialist

Under the Supervision of
Andrew Papineau
Supervisor for the Visually Handicapped
Division for Handicapped Children
Department of Public Instruction
State of Wisconsin

Title VI-B EHA Vision Project

No. 30088

Chapter 89, Laws of 1973, states that, "It is a policy of this state to provide as an integral part of free education, special education sufficient to meet the needs and maximize the capabilities of all children with exceptional educational needs.

The visually impaired are no exception to this law. As State Supervisor for the Visually Handicapped, the philosophy which must prevail is meeting the individual needs of each child. The needs must begin in the home and progress to the various programs available to the visually handicapped. This may be a special program or within the local public school. Whichever deemed to be of greatest benefit can be assisted by the Pre-Cane Orientation and Mobility Outline. This outline only deals with the Basic Skills of orientation and mobility. Teachers become actively involved in teaching these skills whereas advanced skills must be taught by a trained Orientation and Mobility Specialist.

The area of Orientation and Mobility is a vital part of the visually handicapped child's curriculum and through this guide, teachers can gain understanding and preparation in teaching the visually handicapped.

            Andrew Papineau

            State Supervisor for the
            Visually Handicapped

INTRODUCTION

In basic concept formation and most certainly in the development of body image, it is important to remember that the sighted child is able to recall visual images which aid him in the formation of his basic conception of the environment. He therefore perceives a whole image and later breaks the image into parts. The visually impaired child, on the other hand, does not have these visual experiences to recall and must perceive his environment first in parts and then as a whole. It is these steps of discovery that will be outlined here. Hopefully, these parts will be learned in some type of logical progression to later establish realistic conception of the sighted world.

It is recommended that these concepts of basic orientation be taught at the earliest possible time. A specific time should be set aside during each day to work on these exercises, much in the same manner that reading readiness and daily living skills, for example, are taught.

As you read this guide please keep in mind that it does not represent nor was it intended to represent a whole and conclusive pre-cane orientation and mobility guide. It merely represents possible suggestions for you the parents and instructors to base a program if you desire. It should also be pointed out that the ongoing education of the visually impaired child should know no limits.

TABLE OF CONTENTS

UNIT I	
Body Part Identification	1
UNIT II	
Relationship of Body Parts	3
UNIT III	
Objects to Body Parts	4
UNIT IV	
Objects to Objects	5
UNIT V	
Body Image of Others	6
UNIT VI	
Body Expression	7
UNIT VII	
Body Movement (posture)	8
UNIT VIII	
Body Movement (balance)	9
UNIT IX	
Spacial Relationships (size, shape)	10
UNIT X	
Spacial Relationships (textures)	11
UNIT XI	
Auditory Senses	12
UNIT XII	
Orientation and Mobility Outline	13
I. Sighted Guide	
A. Basic Sighted Guide	13
B. Doorways	16
C. Stairways	17
D. Seating	18
II. Protection	
A. Hand and Forearm Techniques	21
B. Trailing	22

TABLE OF CONTENTS (Contd.)

III. Navigation

    A. Direction Taking 24
    B. Measurement 24
    C. Compass Directions 25

IV. Familiarization

    A. Environmental Information 26
    B. Search Patterns 26
    C. Numbering Systems 28

APPENDICES

    A. Suggested Readings 29

    B. Orientation and Mobility Terms 30

    C. Pre-Mobility Check List 32

    D. Evaluation of Orientation and Mobility Skills 34

UNIT I

BODY IMAGE

IDENTIFICATION OF BODY PARTS

It is important to observe and assess the student's developmental level and self-concept before initiating these lessons. This will help to determine his weak areas and to better facilitate the proper program for the child. The assessment may be carried on through observation of behavior both in and out of the classroom. It is important to point out that although a child may be able to identify various parts of his body, it should not be assumed that he also knows how to manipulate one or more of these in conducting simple body movements.

Goal

The child will be able to identify various parts of his body and what each part is used for.

The instructor may wish to concentrate on the following body parts starting with the top of the head and eventually ending with the feet. This list may be abbreviated or extended depending on the child.

head	lips	arms	chest
hair	teeth	elbows	waist
eyes	cheeks	wrists	buttocks
ears	chin	hands	legs
nose	neck	thumb	knees
mouth	shoulders	fingers	ankles
			feet
			toes

A possible alternative to the above may be to start with simple body parts that are related to one area of the body. For example, face: head, ear, nose, mouth, eye, cheek, and chin. The more complex terms may then be introduced later. It should also be pointed out that the average blind child will not grasp this concept generally before the age of 4 or 5.

Suggested Activities

Records - there are a wide variety of body part records available through educational supply companies. One example is The Play and Learn Series, Summit Industries, P.O. Box 415, Highland Park, Illinois.

Games and Puzzles - jig-saw puzzles that illustrate body parts of children. Science models of the body can be useful to show the students the parts of their bodies, while also illustrating the body image of others.

Art - The child lies on a large sheet of paper. His body is then outlined by the instructor or peers. After it is traced (dark marker for the partially sighted and a tracing wheel for the blind) the image is then cut out. Various parts may be added to the picture and displayed in the room.

Finger Plays - the following are two examples that may be used for the teaching of body parts.

    Here are my ears, and here is my nose;
    Here are my fingers, and here are my toes;
    Here are my eyes, both open wide;
    Here is my mouth with my tooth inside.
    And my busy tongue that helps me to speak,
    Here is my chin, and here are my cheeks,
    Here are my hands that help me play,
    And my feet that run about all day.

(Touch each part of the child as names are located)

    My hands upon my head I place
    On my shoulders,
    On my face,
    On my knees, and at my side,
    Then behind me they will hide.
    This I raise them up so high
    Swiftly let my fingers fly,
    Quickly count 1, 2, 3
    And see how quiet they can be.

A good body image screening test is on pp. 219, of <u>Movement</u> and <u>Spacial</u> <u>Awareness</u> <u>in</u> <u>Blind</u> <u>Children</u> <u>and</u> <u>Youth</u> by B. J. Cratty.

UNIT II

RELATIONSHIP OF VARIOUS BODY PARTS

Goal

The student is able to name certain parts of his body in specified positions relative to other named parts of his body.

Concepts:	up	bottom	under	outside
	down	front	over	sideways
	right	back	middle	
	left	near	face	
	top	far	inside	

This list may be abbreviated or expanded upon to suit the child's needs. The instructor may wish to use only the basic terminology at first and then proceed to the more difficult terms.

Rationale - to achieve effective motor behavior, the student must have accurate concepts of body image and spacial orientation.

Suggested Activities

Such activities such as calisthenics with up-down, etc., will be useful. Also songs, musical chairs, or stringed puppets to show body movements.

Demonstrate activities for the children that they may imitate. For some students it may be necessary to shape their arms, hands, etc., for appropriate gestures.

Songs - Hokey Pokey
Looby Loo
Where is Thumbkin

A simple game to emphasize following directions is Simon Says. The two following activities may also be used:

(The child imitates the teacher and classmates.)

1. nose to wrist
2. chin to chest
3. hands to hips
4. ear to hand
5. elbows to stomach
6. toes to nose
7. wrist to ear
8. fingers to leg
9. chin to forearm

10. elbow to leg
11. fingers to shoulders
12. toes to knee
13. fingers to elbow
14. wrist to knees
15. foot to leg
16. hands to toes
17. toes to toes
18. heels to heels

(Emphasis on use of body parts)

I see with my _____
I smell with my _____
I blind with my _____
I talk with my _____
I clap with my _____

I snap my _____
I walk with my _____
I wave with my _____
I shrug my _____
I jump with my _____

UNIT III

RELATIONSHIP OF OBJECTS TO THE BODY

Goal

The student is able to place his whole or specified parts of his body in different positions with respect to a given object.

Concepts:	across	below	close	side
	around	beneath	high	front
	away	beside	low	
	back	between	top	
	backwards	center	bottom	

Suggested Activities

An object such as a small toy bridge or ladder can be used to emphasize the terms introduced here. For example, the child may walk <u>under</u> the ladder, he may climb <u>over</u> the bridge or he may position himself to the <u>left</u> or <u>right</u> of an object. An endless number of objects may be used in the classroom, such as desks, tables, etc.

A good activity for both body part relationships and object to body part relationships is the simple act of dressing. Here special attention may be focused on the <u>arm</u>, for example, as it goes <u>inside</u> the sleeve.

Objects in relation to body planes (the child is seated in a chair with a box).

    Place the box so that it touches <u>side</u>
    Place the box so that it touches <u>front</u> (stomach)
    Place the box so that it touches <u>back</u>
    Place the box so that it touches <u>top</u> of the head
    Place the box so that it touches <u>bottom</u> of foot

(Touch body parts to surroundings)

Head to door	Nose to window
Hands to wall	Ear to table
Elbows to desk	Fingers to puzzle
Head to chair	Stomach to floor
Upper arm to door	Forearm to wall
Knees to floor	Thigh to chair

UNIT IV

ONE OBJECT TO ANOTHER OBJECT

Goal

The student is able to place specified objects in different positions with respect to other given objects.

Concepts:		
above	across	around
away	back	behind
below	beneath	beside
between	bottom	center
close	far	front
higher	inside	left
outside	over	parallel
right	straight	perpendicular
top	under	straight across
underneath		

Suggested Activities

Games and activities may include any of a number of various toys and games on the market that illustrate these concepts.

One very good source for these is Developmental Learning Materials, 3505 N. Ashland Avenue, Chicago, Illinois 60657.

(Using a saucer, glass and spoon)

Place the spoon in _front_ of the saucer.
Place the glass in _back_ of the spoon.
Place the spoon _behind_ the glass.
Place the spoon _over_ the glass.
Place the spoon to the _right_ of the saucer.
Place the saucer _higher_ than the glass.

UNIT V

BODY IMAGE OF OTHERS

Body image of another person and the ability to verbally describe self and others.

Goal

The student will demonstrate the ability to identify the body image of another person and to verbally describe self and others.

Rationale

If the sightless child does not know the nature of space he occupies, the manner which he can move and the names given to his body and its parts, it is unrealistic to expect him to function in space.

Concepts:		
ankle	arm	heel
back	bottom	calf
cheeks	chest	chin
ear	elbow	eye
face	fingernails	foot
forearm	forehead	head
hair	hand	index finger
heel	hip	little finger
knee	knuckles	middle finger
lips	neck	palm
mouth	nose	little finger
ribs	shin	toes
leg	teeth	wrist
tongue	waist	

The student should be expected to identify more complex body parts as compared to the first unit on body image. It is important that he understand that all people have bodies and body parts similar to but in some ways different from their own.

The use of dolls and mannequins may teach the body image of others and at the same time teach that people are of various size relative to others.

UNIT VI

BODY EXPRESSION

Goal

The student will demonstrate the use of proper body expression in a sighted world.

One of the more important aspects of education of the visually handicapped youngster is that of proper body expression techniques. All too often, a blind person will distract others with improper body movements or expressions.

A common misconception by the sighted public is that this body expression is natural for everyone and does not take into consideration that much of this expression is learned through visual observations. It is often, therefore, quite distracting to many if a student does not face them in a conversation, for example.

The following ideas represent areas that may be concentrated on but by no means is thought of as a complete list. Many of these also represent areas where good social sense is stressed and hopefully, brought about.

    Body expression concepts:

    following a person's voice to whom one is speaking or listening with one's eyes

    facing people when speaking or listening to them at a proper distance

    using the correct pitch and intensity of one's voice in social situations

expressing:	happiness	wave
	sorrow	wink
	surprise	point
	shrug	
	nod (yes, no)	

Interrelated with correct body expression is the problem of inappropriate behavior patterns exhibited by some children. This behavior, commonly known as "blindisms" is considered an "act of automatic self-stimulation" to compensate for the lack of stimulation from the outside world. Common "blindisms" are rocking, eye poking, finger snapping and fast head moving.

The child should become aware of these inappropriate behaviors and encouraged to curtail them.

BODY MOVEMENT

Posture

One of the more important aspects of a body movement program is that of proper posture for the child. This is true from the standpoint that the visually impaired child cannot observe what is considered correct posture and ease of body movement as the sighted child does. Also, certain self-protective gestures may appear shortly after walking begins. For example, a toeing-out by the feet may be in part due to a technique of contacting obstacles first with the feet rather than the body. If these abnormalities in gait and posture are allowed to continue it will often be more difficult or, in some cases, impossible to correct later.

Possible areas of concentration:

Correct gait
Correct head carriage
Correct arm and hand position
Correct standing position
Correct setting position

Perhaps the most common display of poor posture is that of dropping the head or carrying it forward of the center line of the body.

It should be the parents or teachers responsibility to encourage correct posture as soon as possible while motivating the child towards good posture. The benefits and adverse effects of good and poor posture should also be pointed out.

Posture is more than standing erectly. It is also maintaining efficiency and grace as the body moves through work and play of a normal day. Finally, the desire must come from within the child before any change will take place.

Suggested Activities

1. Stand and walk with bean bag or book on the head.

2. Walk on the balance board to develop balance and coordination.

3. Use a jointed doll or wire dolls to demonstrate the difference between good and poor posture.

4. Use the student's or instructor's body to demonstrate posture. Let the child feel body position.

5. Make use of straight surfaces or walls to illustrate correct posture.

UNIT VIII

BODY MOVEMENT

Balance and Basic Movement Skills

The following is a partial list of skills that you may wish to concentrate on as the child's skills develops:

roll	skip	dodge	hop
run	walk	jump	gallop
slide	crawl	land	fall

Basic Movement Skills

Walk - alternate transfer of weight from one foot to the other; arms swinging freely in opposition. One foot is always in contact with the floor.

Run - faster than a walk; both feet are off the floor at the highest point.

Jump - take off from one or both feet and land on both feet.

Leap - a run with more elevation and space covered by each step. Body is suspended in the air between each step.

Gallop - a walk and a run with the same foot leading. Back foot is brought up to but not past the front foot on each gallop.

Skip - a quick hop on one foot and a step forward on the other.

Slide - same as a gallop; movement is sideways.

Suggested Activities

(practice activities for balance)

hands   a. raise one hand in the air, then alternate

legs   b. raise one leg in the air, then alternate

           c. raise right legs and left legs alternately

           d. balance on tiptoes and count to ten

           e. stand on one foot to the count of five and then alternate feet

UNIT IX

SPACIAL RELATIONSHIPS

For the blind child, the sense of touch (tactual) serves to organize perception of the shape, size and position of objects in his spacial world. The child relies upon the sense of touch in conjunction with his other remaining senses for informational intake.

Size - Tactual

Goal

The student will demonstrate the ability to use the tactual sense in comparative size and weight.

big	huge	wide
heavy	tiny	narrow
little	long	tall
light	short	great
fat	large	length
thin	small	width
average	half	height
thin	thick	whole

Suggested Activities

There are a limitless amount of activities that may be used here with concentration centered on comparing materials.

    (differences in weight)

full vs. empty
movable vs. immovable
heavy - heavier
light - lighter

Shape - Tactual

The child should recognize the differences in these shapes:

round	cube
square	corner
rectangle	round
triangle	semi-circle
arc	straight

UNIT X

SPACIAL RELATIONSHIPS

Textures - Tactual

The child should be able to recognize the differences and similarities of the following:

rough	dry	slimy
smooth	wet	sticky
soft	coarse	slippery
hard	dull	
damp	sharp	

Textures - Temperatures

hot	cold	chilly
warm	cool	humid
dry	windy	shade

UNIT XI

AUDITORY SENSES (HEARING)

Goal

The student will demonstrate the ability to localize sounds and auditory stimulus.

Areas of concentration:

> *close or further than another sound*
> *direction from which sounds are coming*
> *distance from which sounds are coming*
> *height from which sounds are coming*
> *moving vs. stationary*
> *loud vs. soft*

The importance of stressing auditory skills cannot be minimized. The visually impaired students may utilize auditory skills in the areas of:

1. listening skills

2. communication

3. modes: verbal, written, taped

The child should be made to realize that sounds are all around him, within him, and made by him. He must learn to use these sounds intelligently and pick out the sounds that are of value to him.

UNIT XII

ORIENTATION AND MOBILITY UNIT OUTLINE

I. SIGHTED GUIDE

   A. Basic Sighted Guide

Purpose - To enable the student to utilize environmental clues (auditory, tactual) in conjunction with a sighted guide to promote ease and grace of travel.

      1. Establishing Contact

Procedure -
- a. To make contact with the student, the guide may place his arm in direct contact with the arm of the student, or the student may locate the guide's arm by moving the forearm nearest the guide towards him in a horizontal position until contact is made.
- b. Variations of this technique may include back of hand to back of hand.

Rationale - Establishing contact with a minimum of effort is essential to put the student and guide at ease, thus enhancing the teamwork approach to basic sighted guide travel.

Observations - Although the above techniques are suggested, the guide and student may vary approaches of making contact after working together. Simple auditory clues, "grab a wing" for example, may be sufficient to make contact. The important idea is that both guide and student are comfortable with whatever approach is used and that it works for them.

      2. Position and Grip

Purpose - To allow the student to follow the guide in a safe and comfortable manner that optimizes the tactual and environmental clues given.

Procedure -
- a. The student grasps the guide's arm firmly, immediately above the elbow.
- b. The student's thumb is on the outside of the guide's arm, and the fingers are on the inside of the arm.
- c. The student's arm is flexed at the elbow with the upper arm close to the body.

onale -

rvations -

ose -

edure -

      d. The student should be positioned one half step behind, and to the side of the guide with his shoulder of the guide's arm.

These steps should be followed in order to interpret the guide's body movements, and therefore, the safe and proper path that should be followed. It is important for the student to maintain the position of the upper arm as described especially when turning corners or making turns to avoid moving beyond the protection of the guide.

      a. If the guide's arm is too large for the student to grasp, the curved part of the student's hand between the index finger and thumb may be used to maintain contact with the guide.

      b. When leaving the student, it is best to position him next to an object to be used as a reference point.

      c. It is important that the guide and student work as a team and not just a convenient mode of travel for the student that requires no work on his part. The student should be aware of his responsibilities and the route can be varied to enhance the skills needed for sighted guide travel.

      d. The time taken for the student to acquire these skills will vary with individuals. Different methods for feedback can be implemented and should be used to evaluate progress and remediate skills when applicable.

3. Transferring sides

To enable the student to transfer sides in a manner that minimizes confusion.

      a. The student places his free hand on the guide's arm closest to him and estimates the distance to the guide's arm furthest from him. After making contact with this arm the student places his other hand on the guide's arm in a manner such that his free hand is opposite the guide's arm.

      b. Modification - The student turns at a ninety degree angle and places his free hand on the guide's arm nearest him. Simultaneously he trails the guide's back with his free hand until contact is made with the guide's other arm. As the student changes sides his hands are again switched in a manner such that the student's free hand is opposite the guide while his other hand is grasping the guide's arm.

| | The transfer of sides is helpful in such a situation that the guide could affort better protection to the student if on the opposite side.

4. Narrow Passageways

| | To enable the student to negotiate narrow passageways in a safe and efficient manner.

    a. The guide extends his arm back and to the midline of his body.

    b. The student responds by extending his arm, placing him one full step, and directly behind his guide.

    c. When the guide resumes the normal position, the student will know that the way is clear and he will return to his position.

| | While passing through the narrow opening the student should make certain that he is one full step behind his guide so as not to step on the guide's heels.

5. Accepting or Refusing Aid

| | To enable the student to take charge of the situation when confronted by an inexperienced guide or when the student prefers not to accept aid.

    a. Limp arm - as the student is grasped by the arm to be propelled, he completely relaxes that arm while the body and feet remain stationary.

    b. As the student's arm is grasped to be propelled, his body and feet remain stationary while permitting his arm and elbow to be pushed ahead of the body. With the opposite hand, he reaches across the front of his body and grasps the guide's wrist, pulling his forearm forward. Simultaneously, the student frees his arm and in one motion brings it behind the guide's arm and grasps his elbow.

    a. Some verbal explanation should also accompany this technique so as to demonstrate to the guide what the student desires and to avoid offending the guide when offering assistance.

    b. This technique should be used when the student desires no assistance or when he desires the guide to be in the proper position to offer assistance.

Purpose – To enable the student to negotiate doors in an efficient and safe manner while demonstrating ease and grace.

1. Assisting Guide

Purpose – To enable the student to better complement the team approach to the sighted guide while fulfilling his assignment in smooth negotiation of doors.

Procedure –

a. To push door outward – The guide starts through the door. In moving forward the student simultaneously brings his hand to the modified forearm technique with his palm facing the door. He steps to the edge of the door and catches it with his palm. If the door is to be closed, the student locates the knob on the approach side of the door, grasps it and to close it he steps beyond the edge of the door. He then grasps the opposite knob and reaches back to close the door.

b. To pull in – The relationship and techniques of student and guide are the same as above except that it may be necessary for the guide and student to step back as the door is opened. In closing the door, the student locates the knob and pulls the door closed as he moves through with the guide. If it is a swinging door, the student should extend his arm in a modified forearm position and catch the door with his palm.

c. If the guide and student approach a door where the student is on the side of the guide opposite that side toward which the door opens, the student brings his arm to a modified forearm position to catch the door. If he doesn't make contact within a reasonable period, he then shifts to a position directly behind the guide to pass through the opening.

Observations –

a. There are four possible situations:

- push out towards the right
- pull in towards the right
- push out towards the left
- pull in towards the left

b. For a beginning student the steps are less complex if he is on the side of the guide toward which the door opens. Initially, if there is a particular characteristic with respect to safety, the guide may describe the door or orient the student to it.

16.

2. Carrying Objects

Purpose - To enable the student to switch a load of objects in order to better participate in sighted guide technique of negotiating doorways.

Procedure - The student is introduced to various situations in which he has to release gripping hand to switch objects.

Rationale - This technique is to give the student control of the door after the guide has passed through.

Observations -
a. This exercise should reinforce the importance of participation in sighted guide technique.

b. If both hands are full, it may be necessary to pass through the door shoulder to shoulder with the guide.

C. Stairways

Purpose - To enable the student to negotiate stairs in a safe manner with a minimum of apprehension.

1. Ascending

a. The guide approaches the edge of stairs and pauses when he reaches the stairs. The student is one-half step behind.

Procedure -
b. The student detects the edge of the stairs with his toe and steps up after the guide. As they proceed the student remains one stair step behind the guide.

The stairs should be approached at right angles thus preventing the guide and student from being on the same level.

Observations -
a. The student should be made aware that the leveling of the guide's arm indicates an even surface.

b. The guide should follow the student visually and be prepared to reach across with his free hand and brace the student from a possible fall.

c. The student may check for the step with one foot and ascend with the other in order to maintain good balance.

d. The rail may or may not be used depending on the physical condition of the student.

e. The student should be fully aware of the guide's movements and the team approach utilized.

f. The student may be introduced to the ascending stairs first and the danger should be minimized.

2. Descending

a. The guide approaches the stairs and stops when his foot makes contact with the edge of the stairs with the student one-half step behind.

b. The guide moves forward only after the student has found the edge of the step.

c. The student is advised to maintain correct posture.

d. The student should remain one stair step behind the guide as they proceed down the stairs.

e. When the guide reaches the landing, his arm will level, indicating the foot of the stairs.

The correct position assumed by the student and the skillful instruction of the guide should help to promote safe and flowing approaches to stairs.

a. As the student gains in proficiency, the guide may merely pause before descending the stairs.

b. On spiral stairs the student has more space at the widest part of the stairs.

D. Seating

To enable the student to negotiate within a crowd of seated people with a minimum of cumbersomeness.

1. General Seating

From front of chair --

a. The guide brings the student in contact with the front edge of the chair and may inform him of the proximity of the chair.

edure -

        b. The student steps forward to make contact with the chair using the side of his leg.

        c. The student "clears" the chair by sweeping his hand vertically and horizontally over the back of the seat and chair.

        d. The student squares off with the chair by aligning the back of his legs against the seat of the chair.

        e. The student may grasp the arms of the chair or the side of the seat to anchor the chair and control his weight.

From back of chair --

    The student reaches out to contact the back of the chair. He follows the width of the back with his hand and then proceeds around the chair to the front while maintaining continuous contact with the chair. The "clearing" and seating follows for front chair seating.

onale -

To enable the student to locate the seat with grace and ease attracting the least amount of attention as possible.

        a. The chair is cleared to avoid sitting on objects that might be in the seat.

rvations -

        b. The student may be manuevered up to the chair.

        c. Many characteristics of the chair may be deciphered by simply using the side of the leg, i.e., height, weight, shape, etc.

    2. Auditorium Seating

        a. The guide is to the outside of the aisle as the two proceed for better manueverability.

edure -

        b. The student is left against the arm of the seat as the guide enters the row ahead of the student.

        c. As the guide steps in front of the student and takes the first step sideways, the student grasps the guide's arm nearest him and follows simultaneously, trailing the back of the seats in front of him.

.onale -

rvations -

   d. The student places his leg against the front
      of the chair, clears the seat and sits.

   e. Leaving --

      The guide steps in front of the student.

   f. Elbow to elbow contact is made while side
      stepping out. The student also trails the
      back of the chairs in front of him.

   g. When in aisle, the student turns 180 degrees
      inward or towards the guide until contact is
      made.

   *The chair is cleared for possible objects. The
   student stays close to the chair in front to avoid
   confronting seated patrons.*

   a. The guide tells the student from which direction
      they are entering the auditorium (front, rear,
      side).

   b. The guide decides what side of the aisle to sit
      on before proceeding.

   c. The guide is on the outside of the aisle more
      for manueverability than protection.

   d. The student is positioned at the arm of the
      chair to allow the guide to proceed in front
      of him.

II. PROTECTION

A. Hand and Forearm Techniques

Purpose - To enable the student to travel unaided within a familiar area in a safe and efficient manner through utilization of his limbs which will provide protection and/or tactual information.

1. Upper Hand and Forearm

    Procedure -
    a. The arm is held at shoulder height parallel to the floor, across the front of the body in such a manner that it affords protection approximately an inch wider than the shoulder. The arm is positioned at an 120 degree angle in such a manner that the elbow is bent in an angle slightly larger than a right angle. The palm faces outward with fingers together.

    b. As the student proceeds, the time between the hand and body encounter will allow the person time to react before the body contacts the obstacle.

    Rationale - This technique will enable the student to offer upper body protection in combination with a cane or with lower body protection.

    Observations -
    a. The student should be selective when using this technique in that certain situations, "shooting a gap" in a hallway, for example, may call for upper arm protection while a different situation could merit another form of protection or a combination of techniques for protection.

    b. Initially, the instructor may follow ahead of the student and give positive types of feedback to help instill confidence. The student should also be allowed periodic rest of the arm while learning the technique.

    c. The instructor may initiate various games and puzzles in order to combat boredom within the student and to demonstrate the practicality of the technique to the student. It should also be stated that the games have their limitations in that often the student may lose insight to the principles of mobility and come to consider it as a game rather than a useful skill.

2. Lower Hand and Forearm

edure -
    a. The student brings the hand to the midline in front of the body about 8 inches from the lower groin, without bending his elbow. The palm is inward toward the body with the fingers relaxed to prevent jamming.

    b. As the student proceeds, the time between the encounter of the object with the hand and not the body will allow time to reach.

onale -
This technique should be used when the student has reason to believe that low objects such as desks, for example, may be encountered.

    a. This technique may be modified by slightly stooping the shoulder when objects below the level of fingertips are believed present.

rvations -
    b. The limitations of this procedure may be that low objects are not always detected.

    c. The student should be aware that these techniques are often used simultaneously and with the cane.

    d. The instructor should view the student from several angles to check that the student is demonstrating proper technique.

B. Trailing

ose -
To enable the student to travel independently, locate specific objects, get a parallel line of travel, and tactually discriminate among objects.

    a. The arm is kept straight at the elbow about a foot ahead of the body at a 45 degree angle.

edure -
    b. The body should be approximately a foot from the wall.

    c. The trailing hand is held with the fingers relaxed and the palm facing outward.

    d. Contact is made with the middle joints of the little and ring finger.

onale -
This technique may be used for a limited mode of mobility, tactual discrimination and can help determine the student's place in space.

rvations -

      a. *Trailing may also be used to detect and react to objects.*

      b. *The instructor should emphasize that the hand is at a 45 degree angle to prevent trailing directly beside the student.*

      c. *When the student reaches an opening, he may then use his other protection techniques until the wall is picked up again.*

III. NAVIGATION

A. Direction Taking

Purpose – To enable a student to acquire a line or spacial plane from an object to better facilitate his travel in a straightforward direction.

1. Perpendicular Alignment

Procedure – The student is introduced to establishing a line on an object by situating himself in a perpendicular position with the object.

Rationale – Perpendicular alignment is a helpful method of direction taking when the student desires to proceed at right angles with the object and simultaneously maintain a straight line of travel.

Observations – "Squaring Off" is the act of aligning the student's body at a perpendicular angle to an object for the purpose of acquiring a line of direction.

2. Parallel Alignment

Purpose – The student establishes a line on an object by situating himself in a parallel position with the object.

Rationale – This is a helpful technique when traveling parallel to an object whose surface lines project into space in a line towards the desired direction.

Observations – Trailing a surface may be used to determine one's position in space and to get a parallel line of travel.

B. Measurement

Purpose – To enable the student to relate to his environment in terms of self-awareness in space and familiarization of labels given to measurement by a sighted society.

1. Distance

Procedure – The student is introduced to elements within his environment that are measured in distance.

Rationale – A basic knowledge of measurement in terms of distance is critical to the student in relating to his environment through his self-concept of body image.

                  a. The student should have some idea of shorter measurements before he attempts the longer ones.

rvations -   b. The instructor may mark off distances and have the student walk them off to see if he can judge them correctly.

                  c. Body and body parts can be used in measuring objects.

            2. Time

edure -   The student is introduced to measurement of the span of events which occur in his environment.

rvations -   a. The student should be aware that there are two types of time: actual and personal. Actual time is measured by the clock and personal time is that which is involved in the student's emotional state when he is doing something. For example, a second may seem like an hour when he is bored, or an hour may seem smaller when he is busy.

                  b. The instructor may reinforce the student's concept of time by having him walk until the student feels a certain amount of time has gone by.

       C. Compass Directions

ose -   To enable the student to identify fixed points within his environment as a tool of navigation to better enhance his travel.

edure -   The student is introduced to the fixed points within his environment.

                  a. The student faces a direction (usually North) and is shown that at 90 degree intervals are East, South and West.

rvations -   b. The instructor may label the walls of a room and the sides of desks with compass points.

                  c. Exercises such as pointing to directions and practice turns may be implemented to instill directionality between a student and object.

IV. FAMILIARIZATION

A. Environmental Information

Purpose – To enable the student to utilize his environment through his remaining senses to establish his position and relationship to other significant objects in that environment.

1. Landmarks

Procedure – The student is introduced to elements within his environment that are stationary and are good locators.

Rationale – The good use of landmarks can enhance good travel for the student.

Observations –
a. The student uses any familiar object or tactual clue that is easily recognized and that has a known location in the environment to help compliment his surroundings.

b. Although a landmark may be any of the above it is most often tactual in nature.

c. A reference point is usually a landmark and is fundamental in familiarization.

2. Clues

Procedure – The student is introduced to elements within his environment that are not necessarily stable or unique.

Rationale – Clues are an instant source of information and thus the student's use of them will greatly enhance more efficient travel.

Observations –
a. The student uses any sound, odor, temperature or tactile stimulus effecting the senses and can be readily converted in determining his position or a line of direction.

b. In establishing a student's awareness of surroundings, clues are often more useful than landmarks.

B. Search Patterns

Purpose – To enable the student to gather information from his environment that satisfies his particular needs.

1. Clock Method

   The student uses the pattern of the face on a clock as an imaginary guide to search an object or area.

   This may be an effective method to orient a student who has already mastered clock positions and might readily associate this to familiarization.

   a. The clock method may be modified in that the student "looks down" at the clock or is situated at six o'clock as opposed to being in the center.

   b. An example of a search pattern is:

      1) The student assumes some basic characteristics.

      2) He selects a point of reference.

      3) The size, shape, and basic features are determined.

      4) The student conducts an informational gathering search based on need.

   c. Both the clock and gridline method may be conducted through a sighted individual or the student. Factors such as time and the value of obtainable knowledge should be considered when implementing familiarization procedures.

   d. Familiarization techniques are used to explore a number of environmental settings and are not limited to rooms, buildings and objects.

2. Gridline Method

   The environment is divided into imaginary lines or sections.

   This may be an effective method to orient the student based on his knowledge of simple geometric shapes.

   a. Natural divisions within the environment may be capitalized on by the student using the gridline method.

   b. The use of a reference point and direction takers should be emphasized when introducing these search patterns.

   c. A method of reinforcement for search patterns is locating dropped objects.

C. Numbering Systems

Purpose -
To make the student aware that houses, streets, rooms, etc., are generally numbered in a systematic way. Knowledge of particular systems will enable him to make assumptions regarding a particular location.

Procedure -
The student is exposed to a variety of numbered situations. He is asked to pinpoint various locations based on his knowledge of the particular numbering systems.

Rationale -
A knowledge of numbering systems and their role in environmental spacial arrangements will enhance the student's ability to travel well.

    a. An odd-even sequence often exists.

Evaluation -
    b. Reference points should be established.

    c. Initially, the floor number is usually indicated.

SUGGESTED READINGS

Barraga, Natalie, Barbara Dorward and Peggy Ford, 1973. *Aids for Teaching Basic Concepts of Sensory Development.* Louisville, Kentucky: American Printing House for the Blind.

Body Image Program. Austin, Texas: Texas School for the Blind.

Cratty, Bryang J., 1971, *Movement and Spacial Awareness in Blind Children and Youth.* Springfield, Illinois: Charles C. Thomas.

Lowenfeld, Berthold, 1973, *The Visually Handicapped Child in School.* New York, New York: The John Day Co.

Lydon, William T., and Loretta M. McGraw, 1973, *Concept Development for Visually Handicapped Children.* New York, New York: American Foundation for the Blind.

Pre-Cane Mobility and Orientation Skills for the Blind, 1966. Lansing, Michigan: The Michigan School for the Blind.

Preschool Learning Activities for the Visually Impaired Child. Office of the Superintendent of Public Instruction, State of Illinois

ORIENTATION AND MOBILITY TERMS

1. ORIENTATION: The process of utilizing the remaining senses in establishing one's position and relationship to all other significant objects in one's environment.

2. MOBILITY: The term used to denote the ability to navigate from one's present fixed position to one's desired position in another part of the environment.

3. SIGHTED GUIDE: A blind person lightly grasping a sighted guide's elbow in taking a walk.

4. MOBILITY CONCEPTS TO BE DEVELOPED: North, east, south, west, right, left, right angle, parallel, veering to one side, square corners.

5. CLUE: Any sound, odor, temperature, tactile, stimulus affecting the senses and can be readily converted in determining one's position or line of direction.

6. DOMINANT CLUE: Of the maze of clues that are present, the one that most adequately fulfills all of the informational needs at that moment.

7. INFORMATION POINT: A familiar object, sound, odor, temperature, or tactual clue whose exact location in the environment is known but is more difficult to recognize or perceive than a landmark.

8. LANDMARK: Any familiar object, sound, odor, temperature, or tactual clue, that is easily recognized and that has a known and exact location in the environment.

9. SOUND LOCATIZATION: To determine the exact bearing or line of direction of the source of a sound.

10. RUN: The term used to denote a course or route mapped out and traveled to a given point or objective.

11. TRAILING: The process of using the back of the fingers to follow lightly over a straight surface for one of the following reasons:

    a. to determine one's place in space
    b. to locate specific objectives
    c. to get a parallel line of travel

12. DIRECTION TAKING: The act of getting a line or course from an object or sound to better facilitate traveling in a straight line toward an objective.

13. DIRECTION INDICATORS: Refers to any straight-lined objects whose surface lines when projected into space will give a course or line of travel in a given direction or to an objective.

14. <u>**SQUARING OFF**</u>: The act of aligning and positioning one's body in relation to an object for the purpose of getting a line of direction and establishing a definite position in the environment.

15. <u>**GUIDE LINE**</u>: The border or edge of a sidewalk or grassline.

The terms used here have been developed by the Instructors at Hines Hospital, Maywood, Illinois. These terms are acknowledged by the University as being standard vocabulary in the area of Orientation and Mobility.

PRE-MOBILITY CHECK LIST

1. Subject does *not* have an obvious hearing loss in the right ear? left ear?
2. Subject *does not* have loss of sensation in the feet?
3. Subject *does not* have loss or weakness in the legs?
4. Subject *has normal* flexion in the dominant wrist?
5. Subject *has normal* flexion in dominant elbow?
6. Subject *has* normal range of motion in dominant arm?
7. Subject *can point* directly at a stationary sound in the room. (voice, radio, clock, etc.)
8. Subject *can point* to specific articles of furniture in the room?
9. Subject *can point* straight up with the arm?
10. Subject *can point* straight down with the arm?
11. Subject *can extend* arms straight forward without difficulty?
12. Subject *can place* arms parallel with each other?
13. Subject *can extend* arms straight out to the sides?
14. Subject *can face* instructor as the latter moves around the room while talking?
15. Given *directions*, subject can indicate the relationship to the three other cardinal *compass* directions?
16. **SENSE OF TURNS**

    a. Subject *can execute* a $90°$ turn to the right?
    b. Subject *can execute* a $90°$ turn to the left?
    c. Subject *can execute* a $180°$ turn to the right?
    d. Subject *can execute* a $180°$ turn to the left?
    e. Subject *can execute* a $360°$ turn to the right?
    f. Subject *can execute* a $360°$ turn to the left?

17. **HEAD POSITION**

    a. Subject's head is not forward?
    b. Subject's head is not tilted laterally?
    c. Subject's head is not turned?

18. GAIT

    a. Does not have splayed feet?
    b. Does not have a hitch when walking?
    c. Does not stagger?
    d. Does not have a wide gait?
    e. Does not have a scissors gait?
    f. Does not toe in?
    g. Does not shuffle when walking?

19. Subject can maintain a straight line of direction while walking across a room?

20. Subject maintains balance while walking?

21. Subject can move around the room with ease? (Does not falter in maneuvering around furniture?)

22. Subject can estimate when he has walked approximately 5 feet? 10 feet? 15 feet?

23. Additional comments

    a. Cooperation
    b. Fatigue
    c. Coordination
    d. Activity in last six months

EVALUATION OF ORIENTATION AND MOBILITY SKILLS

(Indoor and Basic)

Name: _____ Age: _____

Date Instruction Began: _____

Date Instruction Ended: _____

Specialist: _____

I. Utilizing a Sighted Guide:

    a. Ability to locate guide's arm -

        NIY   1 Poor   2 Fair   3 Good   4 Very Good   5 Excellent

    b. Ability to use proper grip -

        NIY   1 Poor   2 Fair   3 Good   4 Very Good   5 Excellent

    c. Ability to use proper arm position -

        NIY   1 Poor   2 Fair   3 Good   4 Very Good   5 Excellent

    d. Ability to maintain proper body position -

uced   NIY   1 Poor   2 Fair   3 Good   4 Very Good   5 Excellent

    e. Ability to react to stops and starts -

        NIY   1 Poor   2 Fair   3 Good   4 Very Good   5 Excellent

    f. Ability to keep posture erect while utilizing guide -

        NIY   1 Poor   2 Fair   3 Good   4 Very Good   5 Excellent

    g. Ability to keep a smooth pace with guide -

        NIY   1 Poor   2 Fair   3 Good   4 Very Good   5 Excellent

Name: _____

h. Ability to travel through narrow spaces with guide -

    NIY   1 Poor   2 Fair   3 Good   4 Very Good   5 Excellent

i. Ability to travel through doors (student's side) -

    NIY   1 Poor   2 Fair   3 Good   4 Very Good   5 Excellent

j. Ability to travel through doors (opposite to student) -

    NIY   1 Poor   2 Fair   3 Good   4 Very Good   5 Excellent

k. Ability to open door for guide -

    NIY   1 Poor   2 Fair   3 Good   4 Very Good   5 Excellent

l. Ability to ascent stairs with guide -

    NIY   1 Poor   2 Fair   3 Good   4 Very Good   5 Excellent

m. Ability to descent stairs with guide -

    NIY   1 Poor   2 Fair   3 Good   4 Very Good   5 Excellent

n. Ability to approach chair (at table) and sit down -

    NIY   1 Poor   2 Fair   3 Good   4 Very Good   5 Excellent

o. Ability to approach sofa and sit down -

    NIY   1 Poor   2 Fair   3 Good   4 Very Good   5 Excellent

p. Ability to sit in auditorium/theatre -

    NIY   1 Poor   2 Fair   3 Good   4 Very Good   5 Excellent

q. Ability to seat guide -

    NIY   1 Poor   2 Fair   3 Good   4 Very Good   5 Excellent

Name: _____

Proper Interaction with Public:

a. Ability to solicit assistance -

| NIY | 1 Poor | 2 Fair | 3 Good | 4 Very Good | 5 Excellent |

b. Ability to refuse assistance (Hines Break) -

| NIY | 1 Poor | 2 Fair | 3 Good | 4 Very Good | 5 Excellent |

c. Ability to shake hands -

| NIY | 1 Poor | 2 Fair | 3 Good | 4 Very Good | 5 Excellent |

Protective Techniques:

a. Ability to use upper hand and forearm (left arm) -

| NIY | 1 Poor | 2 Fair | 3 Good | 4 Very Good | 5 Excellent |

b. Ability to use upper hand and forearm (right arm) -

| NIY | 1 Poor | 2 Fair | 3 Good | 4 Very Good | 5 Excellent |

c. Ability to trail effectively with left hand -

| NIY | 1 Poor | 2 Fair | 3 Good | 4 Very Good | 5 Excellent |

d. Ability to trail effectively with right hand -

| NIY | 1 Poor | 2 Fair | 3 Good | 4 Very Good | 5 Excellent |

e. Ability to use lower hand and forearm (left arm) -

| NIY | 1 Poor | 2 Fair | 3 Good | 4 Very Good | 5 Excellent |

f. Ability to use lower hand and forearm (right arm) -

| NIY | 1 Poor | 2 Fair | 3 Good | 4 Very Good | 5 Excellent |

Name: _____

g. Ability to use good judgment for proper use of protective skills -

1	2	3	4	5
NIY	Poor	Fair	Good	Very Good	Excellent

h. Ability to locate handrail when ascending and descending stairs -

1	2	3	4	5
NIY	Poor	Fair	Good	Very Good	Excellent

IV. Establishing Alignment and Position in Space:

   a. Ability to square off -

1	2	3	4	5
NIY	Poor	Fair	Good	Very Good	Excellent

   b. Ability to utilize direction taking -

1	2	3	4	5
NIY	Poor	Fair	Good	Very Good	Excellent

   c. Ability to utilize the relationship of time and distance -

1	2	3	4	5
NIY	Poor	Fair	Good	Very Good	Excellent

   d. Ability to use good judgment for proper use of alignment skills -

1	2	3	4	5
NIY	Poor	Fair	Good	Very Good	Excellent

V. Locating Desired or Dropped ARticles:

   a. Ability to locate on table -

1	2	3	4	5
NIY	Poor	Fair	Good	Very Good	Excellent

   b. Ability to locate on floor or ground -

1	2	3	4	5
NIY	Poor	Fair	Good	Very Good	Excellent

Name: _____

VI. *Familiarization Procedures:*

a. Ability to use part method for room familiarization -

1	2	3	4	5
NIY	Poor	Fair	Good	Very Good	Excellent

b. Ability to use whole method for room familiarization -

1	2	3	4	5
NIY	Poor	Fair	Good	Very Good	Excellent

c. Ability to do building familiarization -

1	2	3	4	5
NIY	Poor	Fair	Good	Very Good	Excellent

d. Ability to do car familiarization -

1	2	3	4	5
NIY	Poor	Fair	Good	Very Good	Excellent

V. CANE TECHNIQUES

A. General Knowledge

Purpose -- To enable the student to discuss briefly the physical make up, uses, limitations and repair of the long cane.

1. Background

   a. The student is given a brief description concerning the development of the cane.

Procedure --

   b. Information on dogs, electronic devices, and other types of canes should be introduced.

Rationale -- The student may demonstrate a background knowledge of the cane that will complement his utilization of cane techniques.

2. Nomenclature

   a. The student is familiarized with the physical make up of the cane.

Procedure --

Rationale -- Since the cane will be used as a mobility aid, it is of great importance that the student be familiar with all parts of the cane and their use.

Observation -- An acceptable method of familiarizing the student with the cane may be to observe construction of the cane.

B. Diagonal Cane Technique

Purpose -- To enable the student to travel in specific environments through utilization of this technique.

Procedure --

a. The students arm is extended at a 45 degree angle (straight, not locked) with the cane positioned diagonally across the body.

b. The crook is positioned outward (opposite the body) with the reminder grip facing the palm when the cane is held in the right hand.

c. The thumb of the student is placed on the grip so that the thumb faces him. The curved fingers of the student face away from the body on the opposite side of the grip.

d. As the student proceeds, the tip is held out and approximately an inch from the ground in such a manner as to afford protection an inch on either side of the students shoulders.

Rationale --

This technique offers good protection from the waist to the chest and allows for greater reaction time between encounter of objects with the cane and touching them with the body.

Observations --

a. When making turns, the cane is brought in towards the body.

b. Smooth and easy turns should be make as opposed to military style.

c. Limitations of this technique include the inability to pick up drop offs and little protection is given from the knees down on one side.

2. Stairways

　a. Ascending -- The student squares off by putting his toes against the first step.

　b. The cane should extend diagonally across in front of the students body with the hand at shoulder height.

Procedure --

　c. The student moves the tip of the cane so that it touches the back of the second or third step based on the size of the student.

　d. As the student proceeds up the steps, the tip will touch the back of each succeeding step.

　e. As the student approaches the top step, the cane will swing free and signal that there are two steps remaining.

Rationale -- This technique for ascending stairs allows for an efficient method of negotiating stairways with a minimum of confusion.

　a. This technique does not allow for obstacles that may be on the opposite side of the cane tip.

Observations --

　b. Students should be proficient in using the cane in either hand.

Procedure --

　a. Descending -- The student contacts the dropoff with his cane and locks it in place, against the back of the first step.

Procedure --	b.	The student moves up to the cane and examines the height and width of the step.
	c.	The cane is held in a diagonal position so that the tip is in front of his opposite foot. He then proceeds down the stairs.
Rationale --		Holding the cane in this manner keeps the tip approximately a step and a half ahead of the student. When the cane contacts the floor, the student knows he has a step and a half before contacting the landing.

C. Touch Technique

Purpose -- To enable the student to travel within his setting with a maximum of protection offered by the long cane.

   1. Basic Touch Technique

   a. The grip is placed in the palm of the hand with the crook facing the ground.

   b. The index finger is placed along the reminder grip and the cane is held with the thumb and middle finger.

Procedure --
   c. The ring and little finger grip the cane allowing the student added balance and control.

   d. The arm is extended from the shoulder to the midline of the body with the elbow straight but not locked.

   e. The cane is arced one inch on either side of the shoulders using wrist action

only. The tip should remain approximately one inch off the ground before it touches on either side at the end of the arc.

ocedure --

f. Rhythm -- as the student proceeds, the cane is clearing the opposite side to which he is stepping. For example, before the student steps out with his left foot, the area is first cleared. As he steps forward, the cane is brought to the right side to clear that area. Therefore the cane is clearing to the opposite side to which the student is stepping and he is always clearing a path one step ahead of him.

tionale --

When demonstrating the touch technique properly, the student maximizes his lower body protection.

servation --

a. When observing this technique, the instructor should constantly check for: position (hand, shoulder, wrist); in-step; arc; light touch; rhythm; limitations.

2. Trailing

ocedure --

The student proceeds with the proper technique touching the wall approximately an inch from the floor at the end of his arc.

tionale --

This technique is used to detect openings in the wall (doorways, hallways) in order to negotiate specific points within his environment.

Observations --	Specific points may be found in a familiar environment or tactual clues utilized with this technique.
	D. Cane Handling
Purpose --	To enable the student to carry and place his cane in a smooth and efficient manner in most instances.
	1. Placement
	a. The cane is placed where it will create a minimum of cumbersomeness and confusion when not in use.
	For example:
Procedure --	1. When using sighted guide, the cane is tucked under the arm so that the crook is against the back of the student's shoulder. The cane is gripped on the shaft approximately 12 inches below the grip.
	2. The cane may also be grasped in a pencil grip in other instances such as transferring sides or ascending stairs.
	3. When seated, the cane may be placed parallel to the seat behind the student's heels or perpendicular to the student at a large table.
Rationale --	The cane is handled with a minimum of confusion and in such a manner as to not attract attention to the student.

Observations --   The student should be aware that
many techniques are offered to
him. His choice depends on the
situation and the method that is
used best by him.

2. Cane Manipulation

   a. From the tucked position,
      the student moves the arm
      forward rapidly in such a
      manner the cane shaft
      passed through the student's
      hand until the cane grip is
      resting in the palm.

   b. The cane is carried in the
      "pencil grip" fashion when
      negotiating stairs sighted
      guide.

Rationale --   This method allows the student to
have the cane ready for use in a
smooth easy manner.

3. Examining Objects

Procedure --   The cane is held in pencil grip
fashion in front of the body
perpendicular to the floor. The
student brings a free hand to
the cane. He then follows the
cane down to the contact point.

For example, if a door is encountered, the cane may be moved
to either side until the door
knob is found.

4. Transferring Sides

Procedure --   a. As the transfer is initiated,
      the cane is brought parallel
      to the guide's body, pencil
      grip fashion.

rocedure --	b. With the free hand, the student trails the back to find the guide's opposite shoulder. c. The cane is then brought against the guide's opposite arm and is held flush in the student's grip hand. d. After the transfer is made, the cane is again tucked under the student's free arm.
ationale --	This technique minimizes confusion and keeps the cane from the path of both student and guide.
bservation --	The instructor may ask the student to recall the earlier method of transferring sides. Adaptation of the cane in this method should then be smoother.

CPSIA information can be obtained
at www.ICGtesting.com
Printed in the USA
BVHW03*1403200418
513992BV00004B/7/P